Diabetes and Me

Diabetes and Me

AN ESSENTIAL GUIDE FOR KIDS AND PARENTS

TEXT BY
KIM CHALONER

ILLUSTRATED BY
NICK BERTOZZI

A Novel Graphic from Hill and Wang
A division of Farrar, Straus and Giroux
New York

Hill and Wang
A division of Farrar, Straus and Giroux
18 West 18th Street, New York 10011

Library of Congress Cataloging-in-Publication Data
Chaloner, Kim, 1970–
    Diabetes and me : an essential guide for kids and parents / written
by Kim Chaloner & illustrated by Nick Bertozzi. — First edition.
        pages   cm
    Includes bibliographical references.
    ISBN 978-0-8090-2819-1 (hardcover) — ISBN 978-0-8090-3871-8 (pbk.) —
ISBN 978-1-4668-4848-1 (ebook)
    1. Diabetes in children—Juvenile literature.   I. Bertozzi, Nick.   II. Title.

RJ420.D5 C42 2013
618.92'4624—dc23
                                                                      2012036543

Designed by Nick Bertozzi

Hill and Wang books may be purchased for educational, business, or
promotional use. For information on bulk purchases, please contact
the Macmillan Corporate and Premium Sales Department at
1-800-221-7945, extension 5442, or write to
specialmarkets@macmillan.com.

www.fsgbooks.com
www.twitter.com/fsgbooks · www.facebook.com/fsgbooks

1 3 5 7 9 10 8 6 4 2

For Christian Blake Chaloner

CONTENTS

PREFACE

When I was diagnosed with Type 1 diabetes at the age of 16, I was already familiar with blood testing, endocrinologists, and preparing for low blood sugar reactions because my younger brother had been diagnosed when he was 7. Back then, I had a little window into diabetes: the whole family went through a typical education program, back when urine testing and refined pork insulin were still a regular part of treatment, and families practiced giving injections by piercing hapless oranges with syringes filled with water. My brother spent many hours learning how to care for his diabetes as well, time he would rather have spent drawing Spider-Man and playing baseball. Little did I know that I would be in his shoes just eight years later. Once diagnosed, I realized that injecting a few oranges with water in order to better understand my brother's routine was only the tip of the iceberg.

Now diabetes is just one part of the mosaic of my life. I am a science teacher, the mother of two daughters, an author, an environmentalist, a school dean, and an avid traveler. I am able to do things today that I never thought would be possible when I was first diagnosed. The landscape for diabetics has changed dramatically since my brother was 7. New technologies and more precise forms of treatment are making this disease more manageable and, in some surprising ways, actually fun to learn how to handle.

Yet with all of this in mind, diabetes is a disease that asks a lot of you, every day. Learning to successfully manage blood sugar is no cakewalk. I'm happy to be a healthy member of the diabetes community, but like other diabetics, I sometimes feel like managing this disease is a full-time job. Without the support of friends and family, it would be impossible. I will be forever grateful for the empathy and kindness my brother showed me. As we grew up together, he continued to teach me, through his attention, care, and advice, that an involved family is an important part of living with diabetes.

When friends suggested that my husband and I write and illustrate a graphic guide to diabetes for newly diagnosed kids, I thought about how much my brother and I would have preferred to approach the mountain of information we both had to learn in a format that made the task less intimidating. I hope that this guide offers kids (as well as the adults in their lives) an entry point to a disease that connects so many of us, and that it sparks conversations as well.

Our intent is to help diabetics and families of diabetics learn how to create healthy routines, explore new and delicious food choices, establish regular exercise as a part of their lives, and develop resilience when it comes to the ups and downs all diabetics encounter. I also hope that the guide encourages further research into diabetes causes and cures.

—*Kim Chaloner*

Diabetes and Me

PART ONE: WHAT IS DIABETES?

6

WARM UP!

9

*FIFA: Fédération Internationale de Football Association.

I'm Erin.

I'm 12, and I'm new to Type 1.

I skate, ski, do gymnastics, yoga, and I LOVE the Sugar Brothers!

My friend Olivia likes Jay, but I like Mick.

He has diabetes too. I wonder how he feels about it.

I'm Dave.

I'm 14 and was diagnosed with Type 2.

How will I keep up with this?

WHAT IS DIABETES?

WHO HAS DIABETES?

People with Type 1 diabetes:
- are not necessarily overweight or inactive
- can be diagnosed from infancy to their late teens
- sometimes have a family member with the disease, but not always

People with Type 2 diabetes:
- are often overweight (but some Type 2 children are not overweight)
- are often inactive
- often have a family history of diabetes

VERONICA
Type 2 diabetic

ALEAH
Prediabetic

Aleah pre-took my fries at lunch.

Next I'll pre-kick your butt in calculus.

No chance.

Prediabetes means that a person's blood sugar levels are higher than normal, but not high enough to be diagnosed as Type 2 diabetes.

FREDERICK BANTING
· 1891–1941
· 1923 Nobel Prize in Physiology or Medicine
· This scientist discovered insulin's function in humans
· Banting used diabetic dogs, giving them insulin shots to show how insulin worked
· Banting received the Military Cross in 1919 for working under enemy fire in World War I
· Banting shared his award money with his lab partner, Dr. Charles Best

FREDERICK SANGER

- 1918-
- 1958 and 1980 Nobel Prize in Chemistry
- Figured out the sequence of the protein insulin, helping doctors begin to learn how to make human insulin for people with diabetes around the world
- Boating enthusiast
- Peace activist
- Declined a knighthood because he didn't like being called "sir"!

If insulin were a mystery language, he discovered the order of the alphabet.

Another Fred!

DOROTHY CROWFOOT HODGKIN

- 1910-1994
- Was born in Egypt and spent many years in Sudan
- Started studying crystals when she was 10!
- In 1969, Dr. Hodgkin discovered the structure of the insulin molecule, using techniques that earned her the Nobel Prize in Chemistry
- Dr. Hodgkin used X-ray crystallography to discover the structure of complicated molecules like insulin and vitamin B_{12}

If insulin were a mystery language, she learned the grammar of the language.

She is one of only 16 women to get the Nobel Prize in one of the sciences.

Your first experience as a diabetic may have been finding out why you felt bad.

When I was diagnosed, my vision was blurry, and I lost a lot of weight.

My visit to the doctor was a tough day.

FROM DR. DOOM TO THE DREAM

TEAM

YOUR PEDIATRICIAN OR INTERNIST

Main Job:
Pediatricians are your first stop for monitoring your growth and health. It is probably your pediatrician who noticed your symptoms.

Years of Training: 10+.

Special Ops:
Keeping the big picture in mind, as well as answering all your parents' questions!

Frequency of Visits:
Once a year, more if illness occurs.

This specialist has known you for a long time and can help your other doctors make sure that they are all "on the same page."

42

YOUR ENDOCRINOLOGIST

Main Job:
Endocrinologists work on endocrine function. That means that they help you observe, manage, and monitor your diabetes. They are special doctors (specialists) who work just on hormone-producing glands like the thyroid, pancreas, and hypothalamus. Every person with diabetes has an endocrinologist. This is your team leader. He or she can also check you over for diabetic complications such as neuropathy, poor circulation, or other symptoms associated with people who have been in poor control for a long time. Keep up with this doctor, and that won't be you.

Years of Training: 10+.

Special Ops:
Knows how many different body systems work together and how messages are transmitting through your body chemically.

Frequency of Visits:
Three to four times a year, more if necessary.

This specialist is your ultimate diabetes expert.

You know it!

YOUR CERTIFIED DIABETES NURSE EDUCATOR (CDE)

Main Job:
Diabetes educators are health care professionals who focus on educating people who have or are at risk of having diabetes. Diabetes educators apply in-depth knowledge and skills in the biological and social sciences, communication, counseling, and education to provide self-management education and training.

Years of Training:
Often 6+. Educators begin by going to nursing school, then many go on to get certified diabetes educator credentials, and some become board certified in advanced diabetes management (BC-ADM).

Special Ops:
Their specialty is making diabetes make sense for you.

Frequency of Visits:
Anytime you are trying new self-care techniques or new equipment.

Hey, Julia!

Is that the new pump?

How's it work?

You have to make an appointment, no peeking!

47

YOUR CERTIFIED NUTRITION SPECIALIST (CNS)

Main Job:
Food is one of the most important parts of managing diabetes. These specialists can help you find the right foods and help you learn to adjust your diet.

Years of Training:
6+. Although nutritionists may specialize in different foods and populations, they usually have a four-year degree in nutrition science, a master's or PhD in nutrition, and additional certification and licensing.

Special Ops:
If you are what you eat, they help you eat the best you can!

Frequency of Visits:
Usually several after diagnosis, then following major changes in diet or weight or new sports routines.

Granola?

Puffs?

Flakes?

Oatmeal?

I can carb-count anything!

YOUR OPHTHALMOLOGIST

Main Job:
Diabetics have to monitor the small capillaries in the backs of their eyes (retinas). These can indicate your overall health and are susceptible to damage due to prolonged high blood sugars. Your ophthalmologist will look for glaucoma, retinopathy, and any other eyeball issues you may have.

Years of Training: 8+.

Special Ops:
No problem checking if you need glasses too!

Frequency of Visits:
Every year.

I have always been afraid of this part of diabetes.

Going to the ophthalmologist relieves my fears.

People with diabetes used to lose their vision as they got older.

Going blind is avoidable if you have good control and regular checkups.

CARING FOR YOUR FEET

People with diabetes have to take special care of their feet.

Over time, your feet can become vulnerable to lower blood flow and loss of feeling, which can lead to diabetic complications.

However, you can avoid this by having a daily foot care routine.

If you detect any changes in your feet that need attention, a podiatrist can help determine how to treat them.

1. Wash your feet every day, with soap and warm water. Make sure you dry your feet well, especially between your toes, and that you keep your nails trimmed. Moisturize your feet well; this helps prevent cracking and dry skin irritation.

2. Check your feet for injuries such as blisters, cuts, or sores. Tell your doctor if you find something wrong.

It's kind of like a massage. I like it!

3. Always change your socks! Take care of your feet by keeping them toasty and clean in well-fitting socks and shoes.

4. Being barefoot can lead to injuries, so be sure to wear shoes, or water shoes, whenever you are out and about. Keep your feet protected by checking shoes for cracks or punctures from rocks and nails.

YOUR EXERCISE PHYSIOLOGIST

Main Job:
Exercise is a critical part of your program. You need a fun, healthy routine in order to keep your health intact. This person will get you from zero to hero in no time.

Years of Training: 8+.

Special Ops:
This specialist can make all the difference in your long-term care if you are planning to be involved in team sports. A fit and active life can keep diabetes complications at bay.

Frequency of Visits: As needed.

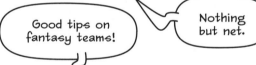

Good tips on fantasy teams!

Nothing but net.

EQUIPMENT #1: KEEPING SCORE

He tests?

She tests?

Always!

Testing often is the KEY to good diabetes care.

A glucometer is your best friend as a diabetic.

It's your hook shot, your lucky pen, your stealth move.

It gives you the most important information you need to stay safe and healthy.

HYPOGLYCEMIA

- Dizziness
- Tingling or numb feelings in your mouth
- Vision problems
- Disorientation
- Weakness
- Headaches

HYPERGLYCEMIA

- Sluggish
- Irritated
- Dehydrated
- Thirsty

When you have eaten foods that have a lot of carbohydrates, your blood sugar can go up.

Hyper means "high," and you know what *glycemia* is now--a measure of sugar.

So, if you have HYPERGLYCEMIA, you have high blood sugar.

LOWS AND HIGHS

People with Type 1 and Type 2 diabetes have made incredible achievements in sports of every kind. Olympic swimmers and ski racers, champion gymnasts and soccer players--people with diabetes are capable, motivated, and competitive in the most prestigious arenas.

Many athletes with diabetes also give back to their communities by working as role models for kids with diabetes or helping organizations raise money for research for a cure.

EQUIPMENT #2: WHAT IS INSULIN, AND WHAT ARE ORAL MEDS?

When I tell people I have diabetes, the first thing they want to talk about are "shots"!

But there is way more to the story than shots.

Marco and I can tell you a thing or two about medication.

People with Type 1 diabetes, like me, can't make insulin.

You put it in as you need it.

Shots, pens, and pumps--they're the only ways.

THE PANCREAS PLAYBOOK

DEAN KAMEN
· 1951–
· Inventor of the insulin pump
· Inventor of the Segway
· Winner of the National Medal of Technology in 2000
· His dad was a cartoonist
· He lives in an ecologically inventive house in the shape of a hexagon
· He is excited about helping kids get into inventing, science, and technology

Whoa!

This is epic!

I want to invent stuff.

Did you know that the technology for the pump came from the Mars *Viking* program at NASA?!

H. G. Wells was a Type 1 too--can he make a time machine?

For people with Type 2 diabetes, oral medications are often prescribed to work alongside exercise and diet recommendations.

Some pills help your body use glucose better, others force your pancreas to make more insulin.

Some pills being studied will be able to block the enzymes that allow you to digest starches, helping your blood sugar to go up slowly rather than "spiking" after a meal.

Sensitizers are pills that make your cells more sensitive to insulin, helping your body to use it more effectively.

Some pills help your pancreas make more insulin right after you eat. These could be star team players in the future!

Some others help increase insulin after you eat, but only need to be taken once a day. Researchers are trying hard to build a "dream team" to support blood sugar control.

Your team is crucial; oral medications can be your MVP.

PART FOUR: FUEL

WHAT IS A CARBOHYDRATE?

93

WHAT ARE FATS?

Fats, or lipids, are an important part of your diet.

They store long-term energy and make up important parts of every cell in your body.

Often, eating fatty foods makes your carbohydrates digest more slowly.

There are many kinds of fat, some healthy, some not. Saturated fat and trans fat are two types that the American Heart Association calls "bad fats."

Think fried.

Think doughnuts.

Think shiny packages covered in TV characters...

Polyunsaturated fat and monounsaturated fat are the better fats.

Olive oils and fats from nuts, lean meats, and fish are good sources.

People need fat, but I learned that if you eat too much, it will get stowed away. Know what I mean?

CARB COUNTING

Carbohydrates, including sugars, need to be accounted for in your diet plan and in your insulin or oral medication dosage.

This is called COUNTING CARBS.

Your diabetes team will help you determine the right amount to eat based on your size and age.

They might ask you to modify the carbs and fats you choose to eat.

Other things you read in a nutrition label are important too.

As you learn about food, you'll find that both children and adults try to keep a lot of nutrients in balance.

Like sodium, in table salt--Mom looks out for that because of high blood pressure.

And cholesterol too.

It's a kind of fat.

As a person with diabetes, you are most concerned about carbs.

But as a whole person, you have a whole body to consider!

Other nutrients like vitamins and minerals are a part of your basic health needs.

But you don't have to get lost in the chemistry, unless that's your thing.

Just a little science can go a long way.

NEW WAYS TO FUEL UP

Most doses of insulin are matched to work with 15 grams of carbohydrates, an easy way to match food and medicine.

You may, for example, take one unit of insulin for every 15 grams of carbohydrates.*

After a while, you get used to recognizing how much that is, like in these examples.

While 15 grams is average, your size and age will determine the number you and your doctor will choose. Please follow your physician's carbohydrate recommendations.

For example, there are about 15 grams of carbohydrates in:

- 1 small apple (4 oz)
- 2/3 cup of plain yogurt
- 2 small cookies
- 1/2 cup ice cream or frozen yogurt
- 1 tablespoon of honey or agave nectar
- 1/2 cup of oatmeal
- 1/2 cup of orzo or couscous
- 1 slice of bread or a small tortilla
- 1/3 cup of pasta or rice
- 4-6 crackers
- 1/2 English muffin
- 1/2 cup of corn or black beans
- 6 fish or chicken nuggets
- 1 cup of tomato soup

*Pump and pen dosages are always determined by your endocrinologist. Please follow your doctor's recommendations at all times.

FOOD MAKEOVER #1: THE BURRITO COMEBACK KID

Please follow all of your physician's recommendations about food choices. Some recommendations from nutritionists or physicians may not match the ones suggested here.

109

111

Oven-Baked Sweet Potato Home Fries

1.   Cut 3 medium-size sweet potatoes into ½-inch-thick strips. Toss with 1 tbsp. olive oil. Put on a nonstick cookie sheet with cooking spray or oil.

2.   Bake at 400 degrees for 15 to 20 minutes, until strips are golden brown on the bottom.

3.   Turn and bake for 15 to 20 minutes more, until strips are golden brown all over.

4.   Add coarse salt and parsley to taste. Makes 2 servings.

I still get french fries. Except now they're orange.

I do like dip.

Curry Dip

1.   Sauté 1/2 cup of chopped scallions in 1 tbsp. butter.

2.   Add 1 tsp. curry powder and mix well. Remove from the heat.

3.   Mix the curried scallions with 1 cup of 2 percent fat yogurt.

4.   Add 1/4 cup of chopped golden raisins. Chill well before serving.

Vinegar is so good.

Veggie Panini Sandwiches

1.   Grill about 1 cup of your favorite veggies, roughly chopped, in olive oil.

2.   On thick, whole wheat panini bread, spread a balsamic-vinegar-and-mustard mix (1 tsp. each) on each side. Before grilling, add 2 thin slices or sprinkle with 1/4 cup grated sharp cheese such as Asiago or Parmesan.

3.   Press in a panini grill or grill like a cheese sandwich.

Please follow all of your physician's recommendations about food choices. Some recommendations from nutritionists or physicians may not match the ones suggested here.

TIME-OUT:
DEALING WITH EMERGENCIES AND FOOD

Earlier we talked about what brings your blood sugar up and down.

You'll try to keep things in the right range, but it is completely normal to have things slip up or down.

With enough testing, you can keep track and respond as needed.

LOWS

Remember that we call lows HYPOGLYCEMIA, meaning low blood sugar.

When you experience symptoms of low blood sugar, your FIRST JOB IS TO TEST YOUR BLOOD.

This is really important.

You don't want to just guess.

Are you okay, Marco?

You may experience symptoms such as dizziness, tingling or numb feelings in your mouth, vision problems, disorientation, weakness, headaches, or irritability.

Always have about 15 grams of fast-acting carbohydrates readily available.

This can be juice, candy, glucose tablets (easy to get at most drug stores), honey, a glass of milk, or any other sugar that is easy to eat.

Fifty?

Oh, mannn...

After eating 15 grams, take a break, and then test again in about 15 minutes.

If your blood level is still low, try another 15 grams.

It can be scary to have low blood sugar.

Remember that treating it immediately is important.

However, don't overtreat lows.

Keep testing and making sure your blood sugar is going up.

If you overeat, then in a short while you will have the opposite problem: high blood sugar.

SEVERE LOWS

TAKING IT TO THE NEXT LEVEL

RUNNING INTERFERENCE

WHAT WILL YOU TRY?

Different sports have different effects on your body and your blood sugar.

ANY activity or sport can be a part of a healthy diabetic plan.

Once you get started, you have passed the biggest hurdle.

Whatever you choose to do, remember--keep moving, mix it up, and reward yourself for a job well done.

SPORT	CALORIC EXPENDITURE IF YOU'RE A 15-YEAR-OLD, 100-POUND, 5-FOOT KID
TAI CHI	151 CALORIES PER HOUR
TENNIS	302 CALORIES PER HOUR
BASKETBALL	352 CALORIES PER HOUR
SKATING	352 CALORIES PER HOUR
SOCCER	453 CALORIES PER HOUR

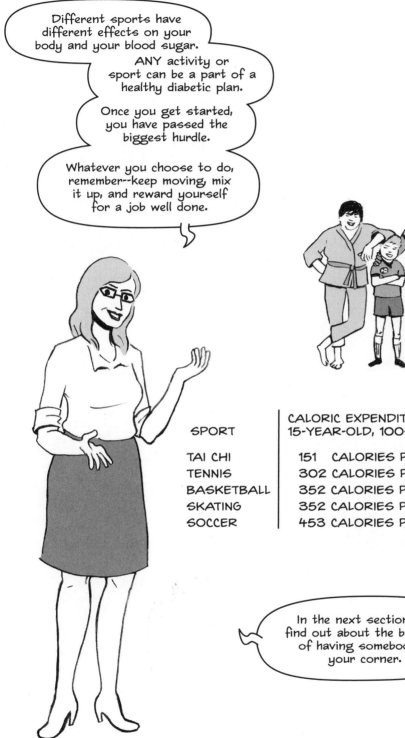

In the next section we'll find out about the benefits of having somebody in your corner.

PART SIX: HUDDLE! TEAM SUPPORT

FANS

SICK DAYS

Sick days are different for people with diabetes.

Illness, especially an infection, can raise your blood sugar.

You should consult with your pediatrician if you have a virus and make sure that you test more often so that you can track changes.

But also rely on help to get through the day.

If your illness includes a loss of appetite or vomiting, you have to be especially careful.

For example, you may have taken a dose of insulin before you realized you were ill, and you may not be able to eat to match your dose.

If you experience low blood sugar during a severe flu, you can hold juice in your mouth and spit it out to raise your blood sugar.

But you MUST contact a doctor and be very wary of severe hypo- or hyperglycemia.

Ughhhhhhh.
I can't even read comics.

KEEPING UP YOUR ROUTINE

MAKING A PUMP ARMBAND/LEG BAND

Materials needed:
- Good scissors
- Needle and thread
- Strong elastic that is at least 2 inches wide and doesn't stretch out easily
- Material for the cover/outside (this works like underwear: subtle colors if you want to hide it, bold colors if you are showing it off)
- Lining material (not entirely necessary but looks nice)
- A fabric pencil
- Your insulin pump or other device

www.instructables.com/id/Insulin-Pump-Garter/#step1

1.

First, measure your pump's dimensions. You will need two pieces of fabric that will wrap around the pump/device as well as create a flap. Don't forget that it's 3-D; add some space horizontally. For my 3½-by-2-inch pump, I measured a rectangle that was 9 inches by 5 inches.

2.

Use this rectangle to cut out two pieces--a lining and a cover.

3.

On the top of your two pieces (wrong sides facing), hem along the edge. If your garter is going to be horizontal, hem the short side; vertical, the long side. If you are using lining material, remember that it should just roll over the edge of the cover, and be careful to sew the edges well so that they won't fray.

4.

Next, measure a piece of elastic around your chosen appendage. If it is your leg, decide where you want the pump to fall and measure the elastic so that it will be snug (not too tight) and have an extra inch or so on each side to be sewn into the garter. You can always trim the extra edge on the inside later on, but it is not easy to adjust the tightness of the elastic once you've sewn it. Therefore, take some time to feel it out before you cut and sew it.

5.

Next, turn the case and lining inside out and fold it up around your actual pump to make sure you have the correct size. Once you've got that lined up, take the pump or device out and put your piece of elastic inside.

6.

Sew the sides several times so that the binding is strong. If you are hand stitching, use a backstitch. If you are machine stitching, go over it three or four times.

7.

That's it. Really, I'm not kidding--you're done. Check the seams, if you must. Decorate. Enjoy!

Diabetes can bring people together in new ways too.

Projects, recipes, charities, and games are just a few of the ways you can make the best of having diabetes.

Once you have the support of your friends, taking more risks and hitting new ground become possible...

GLOSSARY

Basal rate: This is the amount of insulin you are getting constantly from an insulin pump or from a dose of long-acting insulin.

Bolus rate: This is the amount of insulin you take when you eat a full meal, a snack, or any food that contains carbohydrates. Rates vary for each patient, and a physician will recommend dosage to determine what basal/bolus rates you will use.

Cannula: *Cannula* means "little reed" in Latin. It is a flexible tube that is inserted into the body, right under the skin. Insulin flows through the cannula and is absorbed into your blood.

Carbohydrate: Any of a large group of organic compounds found in foods and living tissues including sugars, starch, and cellulose. Carbohydrates are broken down into smaller sugar molecules, which are critical to all body cells that use sugar as their primary energy source. The main form of this sugar is glucose.

Cardio or cardiovascular exercise: Important to your overall health. It will raise your heart rate and help increase blood circulation and circulatory health. Paired with strength training, it adds to your overall fitness and helps your body maintain healthy blood sugar levels.

Diabetic ketoacidosis: Most common in Type 1 diabetics with untreated high blood sugar. Ketoacidosis is detected when the liver breaks down fat and proteins and forms ketones in the blood. This happens when, due to a lack of insulin, the cells do not have glucose available for energy, and begin breaking down other molecules. The glucose normally available also remains in the bloodstream, rather than entering cells with the help of insulin.

Diabetic retinopathy: The damage to the small blood vessels of the retina caused by prolonged high blood sugars. It can lead to blindness. While this damage was more common in diabetics in the past, yearly checkups and careful attention to blood sugar control can prevent eye damage for most diabetics.

Endocrinologist: A person who studies and works in a branch of biology and medicine that deals with the glands and their secretions, called *hormones*. Endocrine glands are important in metabolism, respiration, excretion, movement, reproduction, and the nervous system. Endocrinologists help patients who have too much or too little function in their endocrine glands to maintain their health. For example, because the pancreas, an endocrine gland, does not release insulin in Type 1 diabetics, the endocrinologist helps the patient with insulin injections and regulating blood glucose.

Glucagon: This is a chemical that is normally released by your pancreas to help your liver add glucose to your bloodstream. During a severe hypoglycemic episode, you can inject glucagon into your body so that you can recover from severe hypoglycemia by causing the liver to initiate the release of glucose more quickly than you could digest glucose by eating it.

Glucometer, or glucose meter: A medical device that determines the concentration of glucose in the blood.

Glucose tablets: Fast-acting carbohydrates, sometimes in gel form, that provide diabetics with a quick increase in blood sugar, relieving them from hypoglycemia, or low blood sugar.

Glucose: A type of simple sugar that is an essential energy source to all living beings. It can be linked together in chains that make other sugars, starches, and carbohydrates.

Glycemic index: A system that ranks foods on a scale from 1 to 100 based on their effect on blood sugar levels. A high glycemic index indicates that a food type will cause blood glucose to rise quickly. A low glycemic index indicates that a food type will cause the blood sugar to rise more slowly, but rise nevertheless. Diabetics are encouraged to be cautious of foods with a high glycemic index.

Hemoglobin A1c (HA1c): This test checks the glucose attached to one form of hemoglobin in your blood, Hemoglobin A. It helps doctors determine your average blood sugar over a long period, roughly three months.

Hyperglycemia (or hyperglycæmia) or high blood sugar: The result of either a lack of insulin or insulin resistance following the consumption of carbohydrates. High blood sugar can damage delicate body tissue, so it should be detected early and treated.

Hypoglycemia: Lower than normal blood glucose. The term literally means "less sugar." Low blood sugar can be dangerous, and should be treated with fast-acting glucose immediately.

Insulin: A hormone that regulates the amount of glucose in the body's cells. It is produced by the pancreas, by the beta cells in the islets of Langerhans. The islets of Langerhans are regions of the pancreas that have endocrine cells including those that produce insulin. A lack of insulin, or insulin resistance, can result in diabetes.

Insulin Pump: This is a medical device that delivers insulin to the body through a subcutaneous tube inserted under the skin. Diabetics can deliver insulin that matches the carbohydrates they eat, as well as receive a "basal rate" (or constant flow) of needed insulin.

Ketones: A chemical compound found in the urine of diabetics with high blood sugar, when prolonged high blood sugars and a lack of insulin have caused the body to start breaking down fats and proteins. When ketones are in the blood, they indicate that treatment, usually with insulin, is necessary. You can test your urine for the presence of ketones.

Metabolism: The sum of chemical and physical reactions that a living being uses to maintain life and keep cell function going.

Neuropathy: The name used to describe damage to nerves of the peripheral nervous system that may be caused either by disease or trauma or as a side effect of illness.

Obesity: A word used to describe people who are overweight. Doctors determine how overweight you are based on your BMI, or body mass index, as well as other indicators of your fitness and health. Your physician determines your BMI using your height, weight, and age. If your BMI is above average, you are considered to be obese. While other factors, such as your activity level, are also used to determine your ideal weight, those who are obese or in danger of becoming obese are at a higher risk for Type 2 diabetes.

Ophthalmologist: A specialist in medical and surgical eye problems. An ophthalmologist performs annual eye exams for diabetic patients that include testing the retina for damage due to high blood sugar.

Oral Medication: Refers to any number of oral medications that can help Type 2 diabetics digest carbohydrates. Each medication is designed to do a different job for Type 2 diabetics. Some oral medications help your pancreas release more insulin, while others help the insulin in your body access cells more effectively.

Pancreas: An endocrine and digestive gland, below the stomach, that releases enzymes and hormones into the small intestine. Inside the tissue of the pancreas are the islets of Langerhans, which create and secrete insulin and glucagon.

Reservoir: This is where the liquid insulin is kept in an insulin "pump" in a small cylindrical tube. The pump itself attaches to the reservoir and delivers measured amounts of insulin through a programmed pump.

LIST OF SOURCES

American Diabetes Association. American Diabetes Association website. Accessed July 2011. www.diabetes.org.

———. *Complete Guide to Diabetes: The Ultimate Home Reference from the Diabetes Experts.* 5th ed. Alexandria, VA: American Diabetes Association, 2011.

Behavioral Diabetes Institute. Behavioral Diabetes Institute website. Accessed December 2010. www.behavioraldiabetesinstitute.org.

Colberg, Sheri. *The Diabetes Athlete.* Champaign, IL: Human Kinetics, 2001.

Dean, Laura, MD, and Johanna McEntyre, PhD. *The Genetic Landscape of Diabetes.* Bethesda, MD: National Center for Biotechnology Information, 2004. www.ncbi.nlm.nih.gov.

Diabetes Digital Media Ltd. Diabetes.co.uk. Accessed March 6, 2011. www.diabetes.co.uk.

dLife Foundation. dLife website. Accessed March 2011. www.dlife.com.

Greenberg, Riva. *50 Diabetes Myths That Can Ruin Your Life: And the 50 Diabetes Truths That Can Save It.* Philadelphia: Da Capo Press, 2009.

International Diabetes Federation. "Diabetes Atlas." Accessed January 6, 2012. www.idf.org/diabetesatlas.

JDRF. JDRF website. www.jdrf.org.

Joslin Diabetes Center. "Diabetes Information." Accessed January 2011. www.joslin.org/diabetes_information.html.

Naomi Berrie Diabetes Center. The Naomi Berrie Diabetes Center website. Accessed May 2012. www.nbdiabetes.org.

Nobel Media AB. "Dorothy Crowfoot Hodgkin – Biographical." Accessed February 2011. www.nobelprize.org/nobel_prizes/chemistry/laureates/1964/hodgkin-bio.html.

———. "Frederick G. Banting – Biographical." Accessed February 2011. www.nobelprize.org/nobel_prizes/medicine/laureates/1923/banting-bio.html.

Polonsky, William. *Diabetes Burnout: What to Do When You Can't Take It Anymore.* Alexandria, VA: American Diabetes Association, 1999.

Soltész, Gyula. "Diabetes in Children: Changing Trends in an Emerging Epidemic." *Diabetes Voice* 52 (May 2007): 13–15. Accessed March 13, 2011. www.idf.org/diabetesvoice/files.attachments/article_499_en.pdf.

Vertical Health, LLC. EndocrineWeb. Accessed January 2011. www.endocrineweb.com.

World Diabetes Foundation. World Diabetes Foundation website. Accessed March 19, 2011. www.worlddiabetesfoundation.org.

World Health Organization. "Diabetes." Accessed November 10, 2011. www.who.int/mediacentre/factsheets/fs312/en/index.html.

ACKNOWLEDGMENTS

Many thanks to Amanda Moon, Thomas LeBien, Bob Mecoy, Dean Haspiel, and Daniel Gerstle for their guidance and wise counsel. We are indebted to Dr. Robin Goland of the Naomi Berrie Diabetes Center for providing valuable feedback on the text, and to Dr. Iven Young for providing essential medical advice that has informed my understanding of diabetes. Dr. William Polonsky's writing about the emotional experience of being a diabetic has been a very positive influence, and online writing by Mr. Divabetic, Max Szadek, and Kerri Morrone Sparling of Six Until Me have been a source of motivation and solace.

We would like to thank all the members of our family who have supported Kim in becoming a healthy Type 1 diabetic, and without whom writing this book would not have been possible: Chris Chaloner; Sabina and Ramona Bertozzi; Ted Chaloner; Lydia Walshin; Gretchen, Kurt, and Charlie Haas; and all the Bertozzis—Judith, Edward, Julia, Vanessa, and Allegra. Finally, I would like to thank Dean Kamen, Judith Ambrosini, Jean-Robert Andre, Wendy Small, and Carol Collet for their encouragement and inspiration, and the people at the JDRF for their work in finding a cure.

One of the most empowering things you can do for yourself or your family member is to help support diabetics worldwide by contributing to organizations working toward a cure. We personally recommend the Juvenile Diabetes Research Foundation (www.jdrf.org) and the American Diabetes Association (www.diabetes.org).

A NOTE ABOUT THE AUTHOR

Kim Chaloner is an award-winning middle school science teacher and the dean of community life at an independent private school in Manhattan, where she organizes programs in sustainability, biology, multicultural education, and community service. She was diagnosed with Type 1 diabetes at age sixteen.

A NOTE ABOUT THE ILLUSTRATOR

Nick Bertozzi is an award-winning illustrator and the author of *The Salon* and *Lewis & Clark*. He is the recipient of multiple Harvey Awards and Ignatz Awards, as well as a Xeric Grant. He teaches cartooning at the School of Visual Arts in New York City. He has also taught at the Rhode Island School of Design and the Center for Cartoon Studies in White River Junction, Vermont.

Kim and Nick live with their two daughters in Jackson Heights, New York.